Essential Oils for Your Pets

20 Safe Recipes

Table of Contents

Introduction

First I would like to thank you for downloading *"Essential Oils: Learn About Essential Oils and How You Can Safely Use Them in Treatments for Your Pets' Ailments!"* With the use of essential oils you will be able to treat many conditions that your pet may develop.

Learning how to apply these remedies by using the proper ratio when diluting them will be vital in the results of your treatment. You will learn the common knowledge regarding the variety of essential oils that are available to you and where the oils should be applied, for which ailments. You will be shown how to do this in a simple and easy way using the tips and suggestions offered in this book.

Learning about essential oil treatments can help you to offer your pet a healthy body and immune system. You will be amazed what you can do once you are familiar with the benefits of using essential oils. Reading this book is going to help you and your loved ones to become amazing pet owners and environmentalists.

You will become knowledgeable on the basics of essential oil know-how that will allow you to address many of your pet's ailments and diseases, in a more natural and safe manner. Now it is time to become that great and caring pet owner by learning all about the wonders and benefits behind the use of essential oils for your pets!

Chapter 1. What Are Essential Oils?

What are essential oils? Are they really healthy and important in treating our pets ailments?

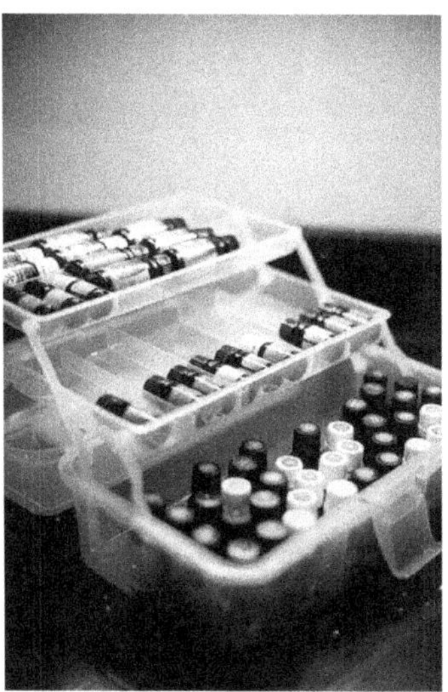

Essential Oils

Essential oils are liquids that are concentrated, they are extracted out of plants during a distillation process. This is often described as the essence of the plant itself, containing within it chemically active components of the plant. Essential oils are basically the very concentrated plant essence.

The name leads us to believe that they are some kind of oil when in fact they are not actually oils, though they do exhibit some of the properties of oils—for example they will float on water. When extracting essential oils it is vital that you know the name of the plant, its origin, the extraction method used and also what the basic chemical components of the essential oil are.

Plants from different parts of the world can have different chemical components, in fact plants that are the same species may have different chemical makeup. Being aware of the distillation process used is important as this process can also have an effect.

The majority of essential oils are extracted from specific parts of the plants such as the twigs, leaves, seed, roots, flowers, peels, citrus, berries, woods, and barks, depending where the essence to be collected is strongest.

Essential oils are so concentrated that it takes large numbers of plants to manufacture essential oils. Because they are so concentrated they are very powerful healers. When it comes to measure the dosage of essential oils you do this in drops not in teaspoons. One small bottle of essential oils can heal a number of ailments, not only in humans but also in pets.

Looking back into our past it is believed that the first people to make use of essential oils was the Egyptians. The Egyptians were well aware of the power of the essential oils using them in many of their healing rituals. Essential oils were viewed as very precious, it was only royals and priests that were allowed to use them.

Other nationalities such as Chinese, Romans and Greeks also used essential oils and herbs as a form of aromatherapy, personal hygiene uses, and various treatments of ailments. Essential oils are still used today by many because of their impressive healing properties.

In many medicinal applications essential oils have been used. These medicinal treatments vary from simple skin treatments to more complex cures; even as a form of alleviation of terminal illnesses. Essential oils medicinal properties have been based around a mix of historical, anecdotal and experimentation evidence. Science has also confirmed some of the claims to be accurate.

Why should you use essential oils? There is many reasons why but here is some of the more crucial reasons listed below.

Essential Oils are a Form of Natural Remedies

Essential oils are naturally grown, collected and obtained by plants. Normally the plants contain some of the most powerful healing components, which are beneficial when it comes to treating ailments.

Essential Oils Are Safe

When correctly applied essential oils will not harm you or your pet. In fact the oils have very few side effects at all. Unfortunately, I cannot say the same when it comes to commercially available medications—many of which cause side effects that can often be just as bad as the symptoms of the ailment they are supposed to be treating. The best thing to do is to do the research and find out what the properties are of the oils and choosing what will be the best ones to use in treating your pet's ailment.

Essential Oils Are Easy to Apply

The way that you will apply the oils to your pets is similar to how you would apply them to yourself. You can have your pet inhale them as you would or dilute them and apply them directly to the skin of the affected area. They will also help your pets to focus and concentrate when you are training them. The oils are also good in treating anxiety issues with your pets.

Essential Oils Are Beneficial

They offer you a natural alternative to dangerous artificial chemical filled or commercially produced remedies, many of which are accompanied with nasty side effects. When using quality essential oils they will be able to help treat ailments such as headaches, memory loss, congestion, pain, nausea and inflammation.

They are also great for stimulating the immune system, helping with killing viruses, fungus, bacteria and other skin ailments. The benefits of essential oils are not just seen in humans, but also in pets. When using the right combination of oils you will be able to create a powerful healing remedy for your pets.

Save Money

Compared to expensive commercially available remedies essential oils are inexpensive. You could even choose to make your own essential oils at home, as the plants that contain the oils can be grown in your own yard.

Chapter 2. The Benefits of Using Essential Oils and How to Apply Them

I am sure that you have heard a lot about essential oils and how they can help humans get over disease and sickness and improve their overall health and well-being. However, many of us were not aware that these healing oils could also be used to treat our pets ailments. In this chapter we will look into some of the benefits that your pets can get from using essential oils as a form of treatment and look at ways that they will work to make your pet feel their best.

Benefits of Using Essential Oils

Their is an assortment of benefits that you will be able to get out of using essential oils in treating your pets ailments. Some of these may include the following:

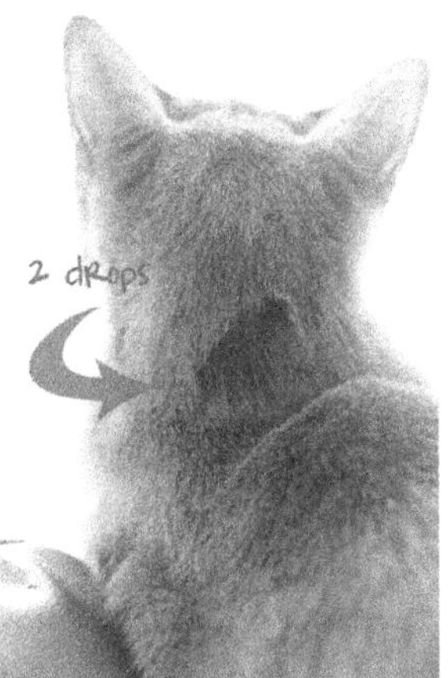

#1: They Are Convenient and Easy to Apply

You may apply them directly on your pet or you may choose to diffuse them in your home. You can use them at anytime and they will be applied in a matter of seconds to your pets.

#2: Easy to Dilute

Just as you would not take the pure form of the oils yourself this is also true when applying them to your pets. The instructions are easy to follow on how to apply the oils to your pets so you will never have to guess.

#3: They Are High in Antioxidants

Your pets can also benefit from having extra antioxidants in their bodies. These are nutrients that are great at getting rid of free radicals, and preventing damage to your pets while strengthening their immune systems.

#4: They Offer Oxygenating Properties

Many essential oils contain extra oxygen molecules. This basically means that they will help to transport different nutrients to the cells in your pets, especially those cells that are being deprived of oxygen. This will allow those cells to heal and become healthier than ever before.

#5: They Can Have an Effect Almost Immediately

Essential oils will not take long to start working for your pets. They will penetrate the skin right away so your pets will feel the effects of them almost instantly after they have been applied.

#6: They Are Safe

Essential oils are safe to use, unlike many other medications that you give your pets. There are some that you should avoid, most of them are going to be really gentle and safe for your pets to use. For the best results make sure that you use them in the correct dose and dilute them correctly.

#7: They Are Organic

You do not need to worry about where essential oils come from because they are organic and safe.

#8: They Improve Health

With the right essential oil health issues can be assisted. Do some research, speak to a vet to find out what essential oils would be best for your pet's ailment.

#9: They Soothe Joints and Muscles

As your pets age, they will have many of the same ailments that humans do. Over time as they age they will develop pain in their joints and muscles. With an essential oil massage, you will be able to reduce this pain so your pets will keep moving strong and happy.

#10: They Soothe Digestion

There will be times when your pet's digestion system is not going to be working at it's best. Essential oils such as peppermint can help with this ailment and have your pet's digestive system up and running like it should.

These are just a few of the benefits that your pet will be able to receive when using essential oils. The oils that you might choose to use for specific benefits may have other benefits that are not listed here. It will be well worth your time to research deeper into each kind of essential oil and study all of the benefits they offer.

How to Use Essential Oils On Your Pets

The most common ways to use essential oils for your pet is through aromatherapy, ingestion, and topical absorption. A great form of therapy to help your pet to calm down is using aromatherapy, this will calm down the whole household. Place the essential oil of your choice into a diffuser and then everyone is going to benefit from the smell and the relaxation that will develop from breathing in that oil.

You may also choose to use topical essential oils for your pets. This method is often used when pets have a particular health issue that would somehow benefit from the use of the essential oil. Using the topical method makes sure that the pet is benefiting from the oil without affecting others. For this method to work on your pet you would have to dilute the essential oil or get it in a cream that has already been prepared and then massage onto the skin of the affected area.

When you use a topical application you are going to need to dilute it according to the weight of your pets. The basic breakdown for either the capsule or the topical use would be a drop for every one hundred pounds of pet's weight. For example, if your dog is 10 pounds you would use 1 drop of essential oil and blend it with at least ten drops of your chosen carrier oil. Then you would take a drop of that mixed solution and give it to your pet. Save the other nine drops to apply on another day.

There is also using ingestion that your pets can be given a pill or essential oil that can be added to their drinking water. If you choose to go with a capsule form you may also try to mix it into their food so they are less likely to notice it there. You must dilute the oil correctly before administering it to your pet. It is as simple and as easy to use essential oils for your pets as it is for yourself. The way that you choose to administer it will often depend on the type of ailment that you are treating and what will work best for your particular needs. You just need to decide which way to administer the oils is best for you and your pet.

Chapter 3. Safe Essential Oils for Cats

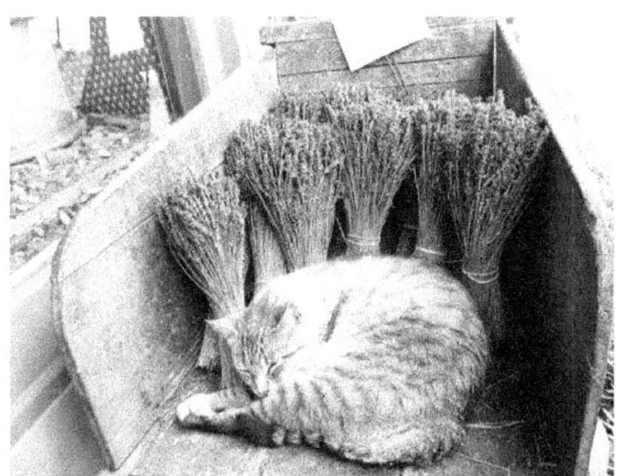

When using essential oils with cats you must be cautious because there are some that are toxic to them. Cats tend to be more delicate and irritable to essential oils, this may be the result of not having the liver enzymes needed to break down and process the chemicals found within the essential oils. This can result in the chemicals accumulating in their bodies and building up to toxic levels.

The membranes of cats' cells are designed in such a way that they can easily absorb potentially harmful chemicals into their blood streams. Cats tend to be very sensitive to clusters of oils with oxygen mixes or compounds such as ketones, phenols, and monoterpenes.

Cats react to the thujone contents of ketones and the carvacrol contents of phenols. They also have negative reactions to oils that contain D-Limonene found in citrus fruits and tea tree oils as well as oils containing Alpha-pinene.

Examples of Ketone are Tansy, Red Cedar Wood, Idaho, Spearmint, Dill, Peppermint, Marigold, Thuja, Hyssop, Sage, Davana, and Yarrow.

Examples of Phenol are Wintergreen, Basil, Clove, Ylang-ylang, Anise, Parsley, Eucalyptus, Nutmeg, Citronella, Marjoram, Cinnamon, Tea Tree, Oregano, Citriodora, Thyme, Mountain Savory, Fennel, Peppermint and Tarragon.

Examples of Alpha Pinene include Dill, Spruce, Rosemary, Eucalyptus, Nutmeg, Verbenone, Douglas Fir, Pine, Cypress, Cistus, Myrtle, Silver Fir, and Juniper. These above mentioned essential oils are not safe to use on cats.

Cats are always spending a great deal of time cleaning themselves. This means that you need to get creative when applying the oil blends. The safest bet is to get the cat to inhale the scent.

If you need to place the oil directly on their skin you will need to place a few drops at the base of their neck, they cannot easily wash there. You may also choose to use the "cone of shame" so that they cannot physically wash themselves. You may also choose to add a few drops to your hands then rub this onto your cat for a lighter application.

I have listed below the essential oils that are safe for cats.

1. Frankincense

This oil is distilled from resin gum that trickles from openings or slits made in the bark of trees. The oil is balsamic, peppery, spicy. This is an oil that is used for calming, properties. It works well in helping treat ailments such as inflammations, anxiety, infections, tumors, snake and insect bites etc.

2. Elemi

It also has an anti-aging agent that helps to soothe sore muscles and nerve pain. It has a nice fresh. It also has antispasmodic and calming effects.

3. Clary Sage

This oil has a grassy, spicy, sharp scent. It helps support the balance of the endocrine system. It helps to provide calming and toning effects amongst other benefits.

4. Geranium

This oil has a leafy, rosy strong scent with a hint of fruit. It is one of the finest grade oils that has a long-lasting scent. It helps in lifting mood, soothes and has balancing effects.

5. Idaho Balsam Fir

This essential oil is beneficial for helping to warm, relax and soothe. It has a nice clean, woody, aroma with balsamic scents. It has effects of security both physically and emotionally, along with a sense of grounding and stability.

6. Helichrysum

This is also referred to as everlasting or straw flowers. It offers treatment for nerve damage, liver issues, bleeding, and wound care. It has regenerative anti-inflammatory, analgesic, and therapeutic effects. It also works well in healing skin irritations, bruises, scars, and other skin conditions.

7. Rosemary

This is known as the herb of tribute. The oil it produces is a colorless strong oil with a camphor scent. It helps to boost the immunity and has strong anti-bacterial effects.

8. Lavender

This is a floral, balsamic, sweet aroma essential oil, that is often blended with other oils. It offers benefits such as helping to relax and calm, soothes, and helps to balance. It is a very safe and gentle oil. It has antibacterial, anti-itch, and nerve calming effects. It can help treat many skin irritations or conditions of cats.

9. Roman Chamomile

This essential oil blends very well with jasmine, bergamot, Neroli, and Clary sage, adding nice warm and fresh addition to the scent when added in small quantities. It is a mild and soothing oil. It has aromatic benefits that include calming and relaxing properties.

These are just some samples of essential oils that you can use on your pets.

Chapter 4. Safe Essential Oils for Dogs

Listed below are some of the safe essential oils that you can use on your dogs, these are oils that are easy to come by and will offer great results. Just remember that you never want to give your pets essential oils internally. They must be diluted to make them safe to use on your pets.

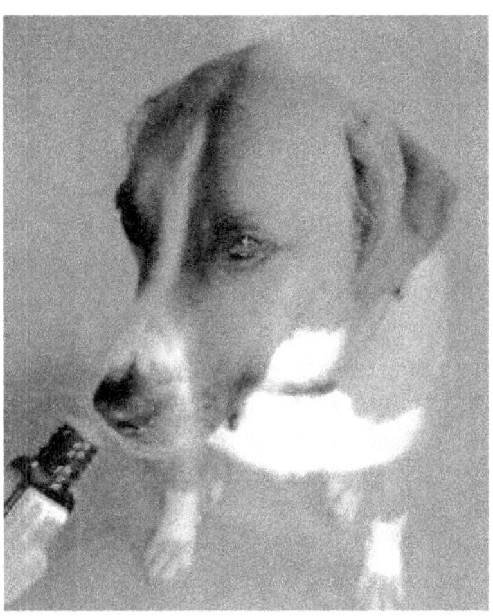

1. Sweet Basil

There are three common types of basil: linalool, exotic, and sweet. Linalool has a sweet, green, floral scent that is often used in perfumery. Exotic basil has a more intense camphor like aroma to it.

For therapeutic use Sweet Basil is the one to use, it has a more herbal fresh, spicy floral aroma to it. It works well with Clary sage, bergamot, lemon and lime. It offers therapeutic effects such as giving feelings of being uplifted and energized, it can work well in an effective tick or flea repellant.

2. Carrot Seed

This oil is extracted from the carrot seed, that gives a woody, earthy, sweet aroma. It offers nourishing, replenishing benefits. It also has anti-inflammatory and antibacterial effects. It is effective in treating flaky and dry skin on dogs and for healing scars.

3. Cassia Bark

This essential oil is also known as Chinese cinnamon, it is believed to be the genuine cinnamon, offering a delicate and sweeter essence than that of other cinnamon. It must be used with caution and be very highly diluted. It offers therapeutic benefits such as giving immune system a boost, and energizing. It is best to inhale this oil rather than applying on skin.

4. Red Cedar Wood

This oil is good at helping you to feel centred and build your inner strength. It is also antibacterial and good to use for skin and coat taming. It will help to repel fleas and help heal skin inflammations.

5. Citronella

There is two types of citronella one is Ceylon and the other is Java. Both types are organic and safe to use. Citronella offers a fresh, grassy, woody fresh aroma. It can help with calming anxious dogs and make and effective insect repellant on pets as well.

6. Clove Bud

This oil is extracted from whole dehydrated clove flower buds. This has a strong fruity-spicy, sweet scent to it. It needs to be applied with extra caution as it can irritate the skin if not diluted properly. If is good at boosting the immunity and helps with respiratory tract ailments.

7. Sweet Fennel

This oil has an earthy anise-like scent with therapeutic benefits of nurturing, restoring and supporting effects. It works great for dogs that suffer from flatulence. It can also boost the circulation and support the respiratory tract as well.

8. Ginger

This oil is warming so it can irritate the skin if not diluted properly. It is good to use on dogs that suffer from motion sickness. It will help to reduce nausea, and is also a good antiviral treatment for your dog.

9. Juniper Berry

This oils is taken from the dried ripe juniper fruit. It has a fresh, woody-pine scent. It is good to use to help detoxify your dog's system if they have eaten something that they should not have or if they have been on medication. It can also help boost the immune system and improve circulation.

10. Lemongrass

This oil is usually extracted from a grass found in Asia. It has a very intense lemony scent, that repels insects. Using it in aromatherapy will help in cleansing and vitalizing. It has antibacterial properties and is also effective as a flea repellant.

These are just some samples of essential oils that you can use on your dogs.

Chapter 5. Essential Oil Recipes for Treating Cats

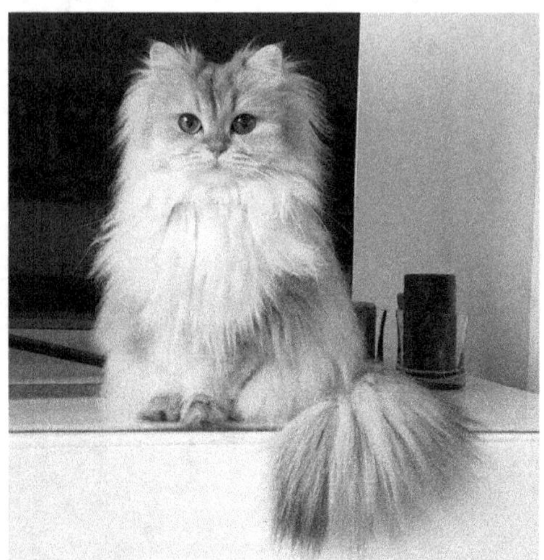

1. Recipe for Treating Depression in Cats

Ingredients:

- 1 drop of jasmine essential oil

- 50 drops of olive oil

Directions:

Mix the olive oil and the jasmine essential oil well then apply this to the back of your cat's neck.

2. Recipe for Courage in Cats

Ingredients:

- 1 drop of yarrow

- 1 drop of sweet pea

- 50 drops of olive oil

Directions:

Mix the oils well then apply this to the back of your cat's neck.

3. Calming Recipe for Cats

Ingredients:

- 1 drop of Calendula essential oil

- 50 drops of olive oil

Directions:

Mix the oils well then apply this to the back of your cat's neck.

4. Recipe for Treating Anxiety in Cats

Ingredients:

- 1 drop of cedarwood essential oil

- 1 drop of lavender essential oil

- 50 drops of olive oil

Directions:

Mix the oils well then apply this to the back of your cat's neck.

5. *Recipe for Flea Treatment for Cats*

Ingredients:

- 1 drop of cedarwood essential oil

- 1 drop of thyme

- 1/2 a cup of olive oil

Directions:

Add the ingredients into a dark glass spray bottle. Shake bottle well to mix contents before each use. Lightly spray your cat with mixture.

6. *Recipe for Flea Treatment for Cats*

Ingredients:

- 1 drop of cedarwood essential oil

- 1 drop of lavender essential oil

- 50 drops of olive oil

Directions:

Blend the ingredients together and then brush the mixture through your cats fur. You may also choose to use a spray mist by adding water to it and gently spray it onto your cat.

7. *Treating Mange in Your Cat*

Ingredients:

- 1 drop of Roman chamomile essential oil
- 1 drop of lavender essential oil
- 50 drops of olive oil

Directions:

Blend these ingredients then add them to your cat shampoo when bathing your cat.

8. *Alleviate Itching for Your Cat*

Ingredients:

- 1 drop of Roman chamomile essential oil
- 1 drop of witch hazel
- 1 drop of rose essential oil
- 1 drop of lavender essential oil
- 50 drops of olive oil

Directions:

Mix ingredients then use a cotton swab to apply to the area of skin that is affected.

9. *Treating Wounds on Your Cat*

Ingredients:

- 1 drop of Roman chamomile essential oil
- 1 drop of rose essential oil
- 1 drop of geranium essential oil
- 1 drop of lavender essential oil
- 50 drops of olive oil

Directions:

Mix the ingredients and apply to the wound with a cotton swab.

10. *Treatment for Cat Ear Sores*

Ingredients:

- 1 drop of lavender essential oil
- 50 drops of olive oil

Directions:

Mix the ingredients then apply using a cotton swab to clean the inside and outside of your cat's ears.

Chapter 6. Essential Oil Recipes for Treating Dogs

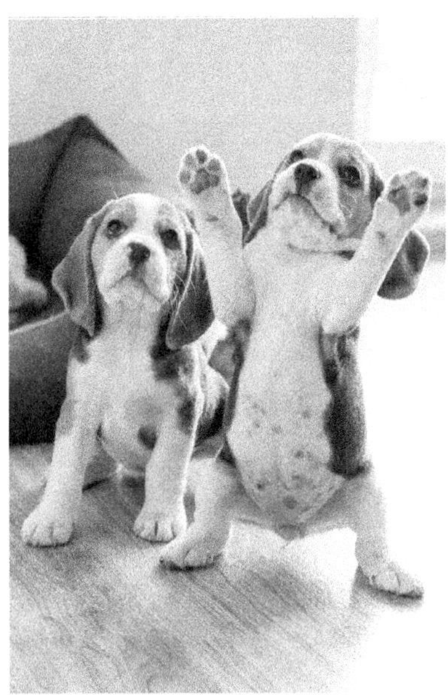

1. Recipe for Cancer Prevention in Dogs

Ingredients:

- 2 drops of tangerine essential oil
- 3 drops of orange essential oil
- 2 drops of grapefruit essential oil
- 150 drops of olive oil

Directions:

Mix the essential oils and olive oil together and then apply the mix to skin areas, that may look unusual, where there might be moles or a change in color or texture of skin.

2. Treat Visible Tumors or Skin Cancer

Ingredients:

- 1 drop of myrrh essential oil

- 2 drops of lavender essential oil

- 3 drops of clove essential oil

- 2 drops of frankincense essential oil

- 150 drops of olive oil

Directions:

Mix the essential oils and olive oil in a glass jar. Apply direct to the cancerous area. Apply frequently throughout the day.

3. Recipe for Toothache and Teething for Dogs

Ingredients:

- 1 drop of tea tree essential oil

- 1 drop of Helichrysum essential oil

- 1 drop of Wintergreen essential oil

- 1 drop of Clove essential oil

Any of the above oils can be used to treat toothache in your dog or for teething puppies along with 50 drops of olive oil. Mix and apply to their jawline or directly on tooth that is bothering them.

4. Recipe for Parasite Oils for Dogs

Ingredients:

You can use one drop of any of the following essential oils together with 50 drops of olive oil:

- fennel essential oil

- thyme essential oil

- clove essential oil

- lemon essential oil

- peppermint essential oil

- ginger essential oil

Directions:

Combine one drop of the essential oil of your choice from the above list with 50 drops of olive oil. Place the mix on the paws this will help to release the internal parasites or you can also place a capsule into your dogs food.

5. Recipe for Splinters in Dogs

Ingredients:

- 1 drop of clove essential oil

- 50 drops of olive oil

Directions:

Mix the oils then apply to area where the splinter is, this will help to draw out the splinter, you will need to continue to apply the mix every 10 minutes or so.

6. *Recipe for Pain Relief for Dogs*

Choose from the essential oils I have listed below using one drop along with 50 drops of olive oil to apply to area that is causing your dog pain.

- Wintergreen essential oil

- Camphor essential oil

- German chamomile essential oil

- Peppermint essential oil

Directions:

Choose an essential oil from the list above and mix it with 50 drops of olive oil and apply to the area that is causing pain to your dog.

7. *Recipe for Arthritis and Rheumatism in Dogs*

Ingredients:

- 8 drops of juniper essential oil

- 8ml of olive oil

- 8 drops of rosemary essential oil

- 8 drops of birch essential oil

Directions:

Fill an 8ml bottle almost to the top with olive oil. Add in your essential oils and shake bottle to blend well. Apply in that morning or at night to reduce pain.

8. *Recipe for Tummy Relief for Dogs*

Ingredients:

- 1 drop of lemongrass essential oil

- 2 drops of peppermint essential oil

- 100 drops of olive oil

Directions:

This can help treat motion sickness or something your dog ate. Just mix the oils and blend well then apply to your dogs stomach area.

9. *Motion Sickness and Vomiting Treatment Recipe for Dogs*

Ingredients:

- 6 drops of ginger essential oil

- 2 tablespoons of almond oil

- 7 drops of peppermint essential oil

Directions:

Mix ingredients in a small glass jar or bottle. Place 1-4 drops of mix on your dog's tongue or you can place a few drops onto a cotton pad and hold this under your dog's nose.

To help with motion sickness when travelling place the cotton pad under your air vent. You may also want to add a drop of lavender oil to help calm your dog.

10. *Lavender Wound Treatment for Dogs*

Ingredients:

- 1 drop lavender essential oil

- 1 tablespoon of water

Directions:

Mix the oil and water in a spray bottle then spray it on the wound. You will need to reapply this treatment often.

Conclusion

I hope that you will find these therapeutic remedies helpful in treating your pets with the amazing help of essential oils and their many medicinal benefits. It will certainly be worth your while to learn how to care for your pets, especially if you are in a situation where you are not able to get the help of a vet.

Knowing these home remedies with the use of essential oils will make you feel much better in being able to care for your beloved pets as best as you can. We all know that the costs of vets can be very expensive if we can treat basic simple ailments with safe home remedies we can also save ourselves a lot of money. Also we can avoid stressing our pets out more and rising their anxiety with a trip to the vets!

Thanks again for downloading my book I appreciate your support of my work. It would really please me to read a review on Amazon of my book by you. Your opinion is important to me!